TO THE READER

Dear reader, have you ever dreamed about losing weight and body fat, and keeping it off FOREVER? Do you want to make sustainable progress – burning fat and gaining muscle? What about having it all at once: quickly losing fat, building muscle, and being physically fit all at the same time?

You might say that doesn't seem realistic, but the information I'm going to share is not based on my fantasies and guesses, but on true scientific facts. I utilised experiments from the latest research as a base for this work – including research from leading medical institutions, not just some commercial magazine or sport nutrition company. The diet plan I'm going to talk about is one that I have continually tested, achieved amazing results with, and really enjoy to follow. This is especially important as an effective workout and nutrition program can only take you so far. It is crucial to feel good whilst following a fitness schedule, as the key ingredient to success is consistency. It may seem to you that "drying out" and feeling good are incompatible, but that's because society has bred the idea that calorie restriction is the only way to slim down.

The plan I suggest is way easier. I am confident in saying that it is the best and most effective plan that has ever existed to stay in shape, be slim, and feel great. I assure you that the genius lies within its simplicity. The following information is going to be by far the best thing you will learn about bodybuilding and fitness this year.

There are lots of useless and even harmful things people do that oppose what is necessary to achieve one's desired results. Excessive food intake is an example. What's the logic behind storing fat when we live in a culture with an abundance of food? Of course, there is no logic, but a more powerful thing leads us this effect – instincts. Instincts force us to do the things that might be of no benefit to us, but are very desirable, especially in the short-term.

Everybody knows by now that if you struggle with extra weight and want to meet a lower desired body weight you must eat less food, cleaner food (i.e. reducing sweet and fat products), and stick to the healthy eating plan for maintainable results as opposed to jumping between temporary 'fad' diets. Despite this, all evidence suggests we continue to practice poor eating habits which leads to continual overeating.

Just a small fraction of people living on our planet are actually implementing the right protocols in regard to what is needed for long-term results, instead of what they desire in the short-term. In fact, I'm not only talking about weight loss. This is true for all the spheres of life. However, as the topic of this material is mainly about burning fat, we're going to stick with talking about healthy eating. Why do some people seem to slim down easily and keep eating right while others can't? Why is there a strong motivation for some people and not for others?

Any goal or achievement requires a successful plan, as well as the right consistency to allow the time to reach such goals. Given, attempting to get rid of subcutaneous fat (i.e. fat under your skin) from months or years of excess eating is a hard task if it is treated as a temporary goal.

There is a whole lot of different methods to losing weight. Some of them seem to work, and some in particular are very effective at producing results. For me, I saw the results of my clients and people I know, gave it much thought, and came to the conclusion

that effectiveness is not the key ingredient to success, but consistency is.

DIETS ARE MEANT TO END, THAT'S THE PROBLEM

This means they give us a temporary result. Most people put up with the uncomfortable idea of significantly reducing the food intake only if they want to reach something valuable in the short-term. This could be a slim down for summer ('beach bod'), a photo shoot, a wedding, a date, a competition; the list is endless.

It is true, we can endure strong restrictions for small periods if we look forward to something in the future that is worthy of such restriction. The problem is, once we start a diet, we also start the countdown waiting for the diet to end. We don't think about our dream body we wanted to get for our goal anymore, as the thought of food seems to override this. We start to remember about how much we used to eat, and how satisfying those treats were at the time. We dream about pizzas we used to order, french fries as a side dish for our lunch, grandma's pies and all the other goodies. We start to wish for this diet to end so we can indulge ourselves with with everything we have been restricted from. So we wait and wait, and when day X comes, we binge.. and binge.. and binge. Finally, all the fat that has been lost from such hard work makes a welcome return. This is the main problem of any diet, and it's the philosophy of these diets that makes us doomed before it has even begun; the temporary restriction of calories.

We want sustainable results in our weight-loss journey, not diets that lead us to temporary progress but long-term dissatisfaction.

Why do some people burn subcutaneous fat easily, while other can't do this at all? That's because those who slim down easily have the appropriate patterns and habits to achieve this.

Let's focus on this fact: to gain appropriate eating patterns, you need to have your own positive experience of changing your body shape.

Consistency in eating right is essential and that's a fact. Nevertheless, once we contemplate that we cannot enjoy a piece of our favorite pizza here and now, we inevitably feel deprived and stressed. If we suggest that the stress is temporary, and we restrict ourselves for a short period of time – It's OK for us, as we can deal with that because we know that it's only for a few months.

However, keeping to a strict diet and exercise plan is different, and subsequently this drives people crazy because they view is as an extremely challenging lifestyle. Everybody knows that it is the right thing to do is attempt to form the correct habits, but people just cannot seem to do it. Why? Because the restrictions are too strong and abrupt. It is true, a person can get used to everything, absolutely everything – but only once enough time is given for the changes to be made step by step. You can form the right habit if you do things GRADUALLY.

This is what you get if you jump into any common-known diet (the ones reducing calorie and nutrient intake):

-       Increase in hunger and appetite - The more extreme the diet is to start off with, the stronger the desire is to eat, as your body is accustomed to a certain amount of calories.

-       Cortisol increase - This is a stress hormone which can break down muscle protein and increase the storage of body fat. It was meant to help us survive from starvation in the wild, but in today's lifestyle it contributes to obesity and can prevent us from losing weight.

-	Insulin inhibition - Cortisol inhibits insulin production. Insulin is a hormone that is produced as a reaction mainly to carbohydrate intake, and also to a slightly lesser extent with protein intake. Generally, the less you eat, the less insulin is produced. More to this, insulin is anticatabolic, so the effect of cortisol is also damaging to muscle protein synthesis.

-	Sugar levels fall - This happens due to the fact that you eat less carbohydrates which would usually convert into glucose and glycogen stores.

-	Leptin levels fall - Leptin is the hormone that inhibits hunger, and makes us feel "full" and satiated. The less fat your cells contain, the less leptin is produced, and this leads to increased levels of hunger.

-	Dopamine levels fall - Dopamine is the hormone of pleasure and satisfaction, as well as motivation. The less dopamine that is produced, the more apathetic you feel.

-	Thyroid hormone levels fall - These hormones are key for optimal metabolism regulation. If the amount of this hormone decreases, your metabolism will slow down.

-	Reproductive sex hormone levels fall - This happens either due to a lack of dietary fat intake, or as a result of insufficient fat stores in the body. Both of these are important for the regulation of cholesterol, which is a raw material used for the production of testosterone.

-        Sympathetic nervous system activity slows down - This system controls the contraction of muscles, blood vessels and internal organs. The sympathetic nervous system is activated by stress reactions. As the tone of the sympathetic nervous system increases, cardiac contractions intensify, their rhythm increases, the rate of excitation in the heart muscle grows, blood vessels become narrower, blood pressure rises, metabolism fastens, blood glucose levels rise, bronchi tubes and pupils widen, secretory activity of the adrenal medulla increases, and the activity within the gastrointestinal tract decreases.

-        Muscle protein balance declines – This happens due to a combination of reduced energy and protein intake. In muscle tissue, there is a constant synthesis and destruction of protein cells, ensuring the renewal and restructuring of muscle tissue. If we want our muscles to grow, we need to ensure that protein synthesis exceeds its breakdown over a set period of time.

So, how does this sound? In all honesty, some of the things above are not as dangerous as they may seem, and may provide some type of benefit, such as a decrease in blood sugar levels. Nevertheless, it is important to keep in mind that this can work only for a short period of time (from a few days to a week).

If we have very low blood sugar levels constantly (for weeks or even months) because of a carbohydrate--free diet, your lipolysis will eventually begin to slow down. In general, I listed the main changes that you should aim to avoid, or at least lessen the effect of.

HOW MUCH AND WHAT KIND OF FAT YOU NEED TO HAVE

Before we start practicing the various nutritional approaches for achieving the desired results, it is beneficial to know the goal weight that we are looking to achieve. From here we can then analyse what is needed to allow us to successfully maintain this weight over time. Specifically, the ideal weight for an individual is going to be in relation to the percentage of fat in our body. How much fat do we really need for health? What is the percentage of body fat we should aim for? There are different points of view and various formulae to find this out. I prefer the following numbers:
• Men = 10-15% fat
• Women = 20-25% fat
If our body fat percentage is within these rates, then our body, hormonal system and metabolism will generally function with no problem in most circumstances. However, excess fat (above the specified standards) may inhibit our ability to build muscle, cause a further storage of body fat, and increase the chances of developing diseases and other health problems. If it were a choice, it is better to have less than the average amount of body fat, not more.

Further, there are three different types of fat inside your body:

- Essential (fat naturally within bone marrow, internal organs, and lipid-rich tissues)
- Subcutaneous (just beneath skin)
- Visceral (surrounding internal organs)

A certain amount of fat is necessary for the optimum functioning of a number of our bodies systems, which we call essential fat. When you meet these minimal necessary requirements by means of food, your body starts storing up subcutaneous fat. This is the type of fat that spoils our appearance and that most people want to get rid of. However, a small amount of subcutaneous fat is desirable to act as a fat reserve when there is a necessity to cover the deficit in essential fat stores. In other words, you need some degree of subcutaneous fat stores to be present for your body to be safe.

Now we come to visceral fat. It consists of brown cells and is located in the abdominal cavity, surrounding your internal organs. Visceral fat is not necessarily bad in totality, as it plays a pivotal task in protecting the internal organs. However, it only requires a small amount of fat for this protection to be made, and further visceral fat stores simply become an excess.

In normal conditions, if a person does not suffer from obesity there is approximately the following proportion:

- Essential/Subcutaneous fat = 90%

- Visceral fat = 10%

However, as the total percentage of body fat increases, the proportionate amount of fat types begins to become skewed. After exceeding a certain limit (men, ~20% fat in the body; women, ~40% fat in the body), the process of depositing visceral fat dramatically accelerates. In practice, this means that a person's paunch grows. Yes, I say paunch, because you can't call it a belly, it's a protruding stomach that you cannot suck in.

Visceral fat does not just spoil your appearance, but it negatively effects the metabolism and significantly changes the endocrine profile. For example, men may suffer from impotence due to a decrease in testosterone levels and an increase in the aromatization of the latter into estrogens (female sex hormones).

FOUR STEPS

It is believed that it takes an average of 21 days to create a useful habit. If you want your brain to get used to something new, you need to do it for about three weeks to form the new neural connection called habit. Once you have this habit of eating right, you can continue doing this with no difficulty in the long run. The whole system of eating right will not seem challenging for you anymore, it will not be depressing. Modern diets are short, and they do not give you the opportunity to get used to them. When you do everything step by step - at first minor restrictions, getting used to them, then progressing to more severe restrictions, getting used to them again, then even more severe restrictions, getting used to them, too - you can achieve a lot!

People usually overestimate what they are capable of in the short term, like "I want to lose weight in a couple of weeks". Likewise, they underestimate their chances in the long term - for example, six months, a year, two years, and they do so in most aspects of life, including nutrition. You need to set the task of developing the right eating habits. Such habits that will help you achieve your dream body and the right percentage of body fat forever, without the need for a short-term diet.

If you want to develop the right eating patterns, you need to consistently make small changes that are easy to implement and gradually and give yourself a very long time to get used to them.

If you stick to that rule, you will be able get used to anything in the future, even accustom yourself to eating the way you eat on a very strict diet. It will be just like a normal healthy eating plan.

I single out four consecutive steps that need to be taken.

You need to move slowly from step to step to form a habit, from simple to complex. Our main task is to learn how to eat effectively. You do not need to lose weight here and now. You need to create conditions for the formation of a good habit to eat less and spend more. This is the basic absolute principle of all diets and systems aimed at getting rid of subcutaneous fat.

The conditions necessary for weight loss can be created in many ways. Here are the ones that are most important and with which we will work:

• Cleaning your fridge from calorie-dense, sugary and fatty foods.

• Reducing time of meals during the day.

• Reducing the amount of food consumed daily.

• Increasing energy consumption around training.

We do everything smoothly in order to give our brain (not the body) time for the formation of a new neural connection. We do not throw all the methods into one big heap, as it is done in traditional diets. Instead, we connect the steps gradually! Month after month. Each step needs time to settle and stay.

Given that the steps are connected gradually and overlap, your brain will have enough time to form the necessary permanent habit.

Step 1: clean your nutrition plan. You can eat as much as you like and whenever you want, but only the right healthy foods.

Step 2: shorten the time of eating during the day. You can eat as much right food as you like, but the time is limited.

Step 3: decrease the amount of food during the day. You continue eating the right food, but there are limits in time and in the amount of food.

Step 4: increase energy consumption. At this stage, we add manipulations with the energy use to the already settled nutrition plan.

It may be that you are already accustomed to one of the steps. For example, you always eat "clean food" (boiled rather than fried, complex carbohydrates rather than simple, lots of fiber and animal protein). Another example: you always eat only until six o'clock in the evening (you are used to a constant reduction of meal time). In the first case, you are already used to the 1st step, and in the second case, to the 2nd step. This means that you can skip them. Please, pay your attention to this: we talk about the situations when you do that constantly. This must be a part of your daily routine without causing any discomfort. If there is discomfort, then let's agree that you still don't have the right habit and you need to go through all the steps according to the general rule for everyone.

Is it OK to "jump over" some of the steps? In theory, it's OK. But in practice, it's not a good idea. Each step is a way to create a gradual deficit. Obviously, some methods can compensate for others. For example, you can eat a non-excessive amount of "dirty food", but this has to be compensated by a shortened eating window during the day. Similarly, if you do not want to reduce the time of eating, you can make up for this by reducing the total amount of food (especially "dirty" food) consumed throughout the day.

It all works. But once again I want to highlight that our main task is not to lose weight, but to form the right habit (a new neural connection). So you can really win in a short time (dry out in a couple of months), but you lose in the long run (for life) because you did not create the right habit.

If you've already been on a diet for a couple of months, you may worry about the 1st step. I understand perfectly well what is bothering you in this case. You do not want to return to that level, because you are afraid to put on fat and lose what you have achieved, as it's said that at the first stage you can eat any "good" products without any restrictions. My answer is still the same - you need a permanent habit, not a one-time drying out with a temporary result.

Moreover, I assure you that if you start making the right food choice after your diet, then your fat loss will be completely different from what you expect, and further fat burning will be easier because leptin, blood sugar and insulin levels will recover.

People are usually afraid to give up diets because this usually means a significant increase in fat due to the unlimited consumption of junk and sugary food. Although if people ate the "right" food after a diet, then their shape would not as compromised compared to prior experiences. Unfortunately, hardly anyone can continue clean eating after a diet is over.

Healthy Eating

There are lots of very different views on healthy eating. What foods can we eat, which eating habits are beneficial for us and which are harmful? Our genetics are dependent upon what our ancestors ate for hundreds, thousands, millions of years. We must eat the food that our body was programmed for by our past and by our origin; eat less refined and sugary foods, cereals - something that appeared recently and something that our body is not ready for. How did our ancestors eat? It is clear that they did not have such an abundance of carbohydrates as we have. There used to be no pasta, no bread, no cookies.

Once agriculture appeared, we began to produce and consume an excess amount of food. Our modern culture is one of food profusion. Throughout our history, people always had a lack of food, they had to make a conscious effort to earn it. We were limited in eating and did not have the opportunity to eat as often and as much compared to todays standards.

This is one of the key reasons why there is a modern day trend for unhealthy eating habits, as the abundance of food availability has led to increased food consumption. With limited time access to food and without the free choice to access food at any time, this once led to more food restrictions and subsequently healthier eating habits.

A long time ago, there were not as many people who suffered from diabetes, for example. That's because people used to eat less frequently and with reduced portion sizes. Due to this, our body was adapted to infrequent nutrient intakes, with a much improved insulin sensitivity when nutrients were being consumed.

Nowadays people's sensitivity to carbohydrates decreases, with insulin sensitivity also being negatively affected, which influences the function of our cells; thus insulin resistance develops.

Mankind has invented a lot of cheap food recently. However, it's said that "There is no such thing as a free lunch" – everything comes at a price. We received food in vast quantities and in return we lost its quality. Certainly, the evolution continues and our body is trying to adjust to the surrounding conditions (food that is always available). But this process is very long, dragged on for hundreds of thousands of years.

Most of the food from our daily nutrition is not suitable for our body because it is still only set up for the food that was available in the Stone Age.

Old food products are more natural for our body and therefore lead us to better health. Many modern foods are harmful to your body, because our body has not yet had time to adapt to these new products.

Products from risk groups:

- cereals (became popular only in the 17th century, so this is a new product for us)
- milk and dairy products (milk contains lactose - not all adults have enzymes that can help to digest it)
- meat (we now consume fatty meat of animals that live on farms. Our ancestors ate meat that was tough, dry and lean)
- alcohol (this is a poison, a chemical element that destroys your system. The caloric content of alcohol is very high – 7kcal per gram)
- oils (trans fats are present in almost all types of oil now. Trans fats completely disrupt the metabolic processes in your body)
- sugar (previously there were no processed sugars, only natural honey or fruit).

The list is really is endless (additives, preservatives, soda, fast food...). Today our food ration consists predominantly of high-calorie foods rich in fats, but with a low density of micronutrients and high-quality proteins.

The natural diet is quite the opposite; a large volume of food, access to high-quality proteins, a reduced caloric content (a lot of fiber, fruits and vegetables), a small yet sufficient amount of fat, with no cereals, dairy products, or alcohol.

I do not want to convince you that you cannot drink milk at all, for example, or that you cannot eat bread. Given, our unique and extraordinary digestive system allows us to digest many different foods, however this does not equate to optimal functioning and health. I want you to adjust your diet more sensibly.

Most of the carbohydrates in your diet should come from vegetables and fruits. The main reason for this is because they contain a lot of fiber. You can eat grains as well - rice and buckwheat.

It is undesirable to use cereal products - pasta, buns, bread, dumplings or any other dishes made with cereal flour, as they contain minimal amounts of dietary fiber.

Protein should be mainly consumed from food of animal origin, ideally with as little amount of fat as possible. This can include lean meat, chicken (breast), fish, and eggs. These are the best sources of protein for our body.

Eggs are a natural product that has the greatest bioavailability value (accepted as 100), meaning we efficiently digest and absorb this type of protein. In fact, our ancestors began using this product a very long time ago as they realised its beneficial effects on the body. Although this is theoretical, this is likely one of the reasons why our digestive system is absolutely adjusted to this food.

Chicken (white meat - breast) is also low fat product. In this regard, chicken meat is biologically similar to the meat that our ancestors ate, and our bodies seem to respond to this food source well.

Most sources of fish are also lean quality protein sources, in addition to being viable sources of phosphorus and essential fatty acids that are necessary to optimise our metabolism and the cholesterol level in our body. Some types of oily fish such as salmon a fish contain more fat, but they are even richer in omega fatty acids – omega-3, omega-6.

In my own top meat chart, beef comes first, then lamb, and then pork. From all the evidence I have seen, this seems to be the right order. In general, the less fat the meat contains, the better it is for our body. Overall, you cannot beat beef for a good source of protein, as it has a high-quality amino acid composition, specifically in regard to leucine which is the essential amino acid responsible for initiating muscle protein synthesis.

I really recommend you to be more careful with dairy products. I know a lot of people who seem to drink milk with no problem, although even these people tend to feel better once they cut out dairy products; increased performance capability, and improved power. Try it, maybe it will work for you too.

You have to make a choice what is more important for you – eating something delicious or getting benefits for your body, despite the limitations needed to achieve the desired result.

People should be ready to sacrifice something if they want to receive something. The bigger prize you want to receive, the more sacrifices you have to prepare for.

This doesn't mean you have to cut out everything you were used to all at once. Just try not to eat bad food constantly. If you love fried potatoes, you may allow for some flexibility to have it once or twice in a week, but such a meal should act as the exception, not your rule.

Step 1.

On the first step, you will have no limits about the time you eat and how much food you eat. The only change you have to make is to actively push the healthy/unhealthy food balance towards the right foods. You can choose some of the things you usually eat, but ensure that there are more healthy products than junk food in your shopping basket.

What food is the most harmful to your body? Two things:

- sugary food (carbohydrates with a high glycemic index)

- fatty food (foods with a high percentage of fat)

You should gradually limit products from these categories on the first stage. These foods give you a lot of extra unnecessary calories, known as "empty calories". Sweet foods tend to increase insulin which slows down fat burning and signals the accumulation of excess fat into stored body fat. Meanwhile, excess fatty food tends to easily accumulate to an excess of energy as it contains over double the amount of calories per gram compared to carbohydrates and protein (1g/0.035oz of fat is ~9 Kcal, and 1g/0.035oz of proteins and carbohydrates is ~4 Kcal).

Moreover, sweets quickly lead us to sharp jumps in insulin concentrations, a transport hormone that instantly takes energy from food to the right places (muscles, subcutaneous fat, etc.). Due to this, this means that you will inevitably feel hungry again quickly after you eat and you will begin to binge on food (leading to an excess of calories). If I had to choose a less harmful product from this list of two "bad" options, then I would choose fat.

Here are the foods you should try to avoid:

- Sugar

- Pastry

- Carbonated soft drinks

- Sweet fruits (such as grapes)

- Chocolate bars

- Chips, Crackers, Popcorn, Corn flakes, waffles

- White bread and its derivatives

- French fries

- Noodles and pasta

- Pelmeni and vareniki (food popular in Slavic culture, made of meat and dough)

- White (sticky) rice

And here's the list of fatty foods that you need to clean your diet from:

- Mayonnaise

- Margarine

- Butter

- Melted fat

- Melted butter

- Pork

- Salo (popular in Slavic culture, a piece of salted, smoked and aged fatback)

- Ducks and geese meat

- Sausages

- Ham

- Canned food

Please note, do not try to cut out fats or carbohydrates completely from your routinediet. First, it will get on your nerves (discomfort will interfere with the formation of a useful eating habit). Secondly, it will begin to create an imbalance in your system, which will lead to a breakdown in health sooner or later. Our body needs all three nutrients: proteins, fats and carbohydrates.

What carbohydrates we should eat: `

- Buckwheat

- Wild (black) rice, red rice

- Brown (basmati) rice

- Whole wheat bread

- Beans and lentils

- Sprouted wheat grains

- Oatmeal

- Pasta from durum wheat - "aldente" (cooked, but still a bit hard inside)

- Fiber (vegetables: tomatoes, cucumbers, broccoli, cabbage, garlic, lettuce, etc.)

Protein is the most important nutrient for us. Why? Because it is not sweet (so it hardly raises insulin) and not fatty (few calories). It also contains the ideal properties for health as well as for fat loss. In addition, our body is basically a protein structure and therefore needs a sufficient amount of a good protein of animal origin as a raw material.

What kind of proteins do we eat:

- Chicken

- Turkey

- Veal

- Beef

- Lamb

- Horsemeat

- Eggs

- Fish

- Fish caviar, crab, shrimp

- Nuts

- Cottage cheese

For our daily goals, we should eat 2g (0.07oz) of protein for each kilo of our bodyweight (each 2.2lb). These numbers are typical for fitness-based goals. For example, if you weigh 90kg (198lb), then you need to receive about 180 grams (6.35oz) of protein of animal origin each day. At the first stage, this information is not very important to you, but it will be necessary at the 3rd one. I decided to ease you into things gradually, so that you know what will happen next. Now your task is to train yourself to eat "good" foods. Focus on cooked meals with protein, vegetables and complex carbohydrates.

50g (1.76oz) of protein per meal – is it a lot or not much? This is, for example, 250g of chicken (8.8oz) or 8 whole eggs. I don't recommend you to scrupulously count calories. Just try to make sure that there is mostly protein and fiber on your plate. Carbohydrates and good fats should occupy a very small part of your plate (<25%).

We need to eat more protein not only because it is ideal for fat burning (it contains few calories and raises insulin to a lesser extent than carbohydrates), but also because a deficit in energy intake requires a proportionate increase in protein intake. In other words, the protein compensates for the reduced energy intake when you eat right which is ideal for retaining or building muscle mass.

Very often people significantly limit the intake of carbohydrates when they are on highly effective diets, and so they have to proportionately raise the intake of protein to 3g per kilo of body weight (0.1oz per 2.2lb). Why so much? Carbohydrate is glucose that is consumed as energy. The problem is that your brain needs about 100g of glucose (3.5oz) per day for normal functioning.

If a person on a diet consumes less than 100g (3.5oz) of carbohydrates, then the body starts to use the restored glycogen (glucose) for maintaining brain functioning. Certainly, this storage is limited and after a few days it ends. In such critical conditions, your body starts using emergency ways of synthesising glucose from other sources:

- Alanine (amino acid from muscles - liver - synthesis of pyruvate and glucose)

- Glutamine (amino acid from muscle - kidney - synthesis of glucose)

- Glycerol (hydrolysis of fat stores)

- Lactate / Pyruvate (a by-product of anaerobic glycolysis - gluconeogenesis)

What does all of this mean? This means that your body starts "eating" muscles in order to provide the brain with glucose. On such a low-carbohydrate diet, blood concentrations of alanine, glutamine and BCAA's are significantly increased. In other words, with restriction of carbohydrates (which is typical for any diet), the need for protein increases. If you eat a lot of carbohydrates, then your body does not need a require as much protein (1.5g per kg – 0.05oz per 2.2lb - of body will be enough). However, if you remove carbohydrates completely or partially, then you need to raise the protein to 2-3 g for each kilo of body weight (0.07 – 0.1oz per 2.2lb).

In terms of this diet, we will not deliberately reduce the intake of carbohydrates to critical numbers, so we won't need too much protein. The intake of high-quality protein food should be increased (2g per kg – 0.07oz per 2.2lb) when drawing up a "good" food plan. Such a diet plan assumes the decrease in the amount of carbohydrates in the future.

A few words about the "benefit" of fruit.

Since we are talking about sweets and carbohydrates, we need to mention fruit. Traditionally, you hear that you cannot allow fat and sweet foods on a diet, but you can have fruit in any amount since they are rich in fiber. Unfortunately, that is not true. Excessive consumption of fruit (especially sweet) can completely block fat burning capabilities.

Fruits contains a simple sugar - fructose. People think this sugar is safer compared to glucose. Alas, this is a mistake. Fructose can significantly damage your diet and its consumption needs to be seriously regulated. If daily intake is more than 50g (1.76oz) per day, the excess fructose starts to be converted into subcutaneous fat.

This being said, an excess quantity of complex carbohydrates can also be turned into fat if glycogen stores are fully stocked in the muscles and liver. However, if we are talking about fructose, then we do not need such a large amount of this sugar for the same negative effect to occur.

It is true that fructose can be stored as glycogen, but only in your liver and not in the muscles. This is an extra reason not to eat a lot of sweet fruit for those of you who spend hours at the gym. After all, in this case we are even more interested in the energy stores within the muscles (muscle glycogen) and their 'fullness'.

Here are three simple rules for food intake that can really boost your fat loss:

1. Chew hard food - The harder the food you eat is, the more you have to work your jaws, so the food comes slowly and evenly. This process will give you the sense of fullness, so try to give preference to solid food.
2. Don't drink cocktails - The fact is that cocktails immediately give you a lot of calories with a very small feeling of satiety. In fact, high-calorie drinks increase appetite, instead of reducing it. It's OK to drink pure amino acid cocktails in a moderate amount, but it's not advisable to drink gainer shakes or protein mixtures for most people.
3. Ready meals - In bodybuilding, you should eat small portions frequently to gain muscle (6 times a day) as this allows muscle protein synthesis to be more consistently elevated throughout the day. However, according to my observations, more traditional food servings (3 times a day) in larger portions gives a better sense of satiety than smaller, more frequent meals, after which you are constantly hungry.

At step 1, it is necessary to clean your food basket in such a way that you eat more healthy foods, and less junk food. However, we don't limit the quantity – eat as much as necessary for you. I'm not saying that you have to completely remove your favourite "wrong" foods. You just should shift the balance towards the right foods which you have just learnt about. You may change this proportion in a period which is suitable for you and your lifestyle. There's no need to do it in three weeks - three months is absolutely OK if necessary. We do not care how fast we go, it's not a diet, it's a lifestyle. All we care about is to move in the right direction.

If it takes a year to develop the right habits this is not a problem. It will mean that in a year you'll have the right diet for your life. You do not have to suffer from temporary challenging diets, you just have to get used to the right one which suits you personally.

Therefore, we try to reduce the amount of sweets and fatty foods. Instead, we eat more fiber, green vegetables, boiled eggs, meat and fish to replace the previous 'junk'. More right foods - less junk, sugary and fatty food.

Once we are used to it, we go to the second step.

Step 2.

So what needs to be in place to be able to proceed to the second step? Quite simply, you should be eating healthy, high-quality foods (animal protein, fiber, complex carbohydrates and polyunsaturated fats) on a regular basis and with no effort, and no suffering. By this time, you should not be consuming unhealthy foods (sweet and fatty) on a regular basis.

The main idea of the second step is that we begin to create a slight deficit of incoming energy (calories) by reducing the time we allow ourselves to eat during the day – food window. Remember, there is only one legitimate method to getting rid of subcutaneous fat, and this is to create an energy deficit. This means that you should consume less energy than you expend every day. All other methods and schemes that you may have heard of are just different ways to implement this principle, as they are all based around some form of restriction.

Our body has been used to a lack of food for millions of years. In todays times where energy intake is at an all-time high this natural balance has been violated, so in order to return the balance, you have to return to the habits that our body is programmed towards. Creating an energy deficit will allow the body to begin working well again, primarily by increasing the sensitivity to insulin. This means you will start to use food more efficiently and a number of enzymes that are responsible for fat burning will be activated.

Usually people eat from morning till night. People wake up – eat, and it continues all day long. There are also people who follow a split food diet - the so-called bodybuilding approach - that says that it is necessary to boost your metabolism in order to dry out and other nonsense. In fact, this does not happen. On such a diet you will maintain a high insulin concentration throughout the day, and when insulin is produced you cannot burn fat.

A lot of scientific experiments and scientific discoveries happen each year, and recently there has been a trend to analyse the effects of fasting. Now we know that infrequent meals leads to low insulin in the blood, whereas frequent meals causes high insulin levels which slow down fat loss. Considering hunger as our enemy, this method allows us not to get too hungry. Our digestive system, instead of getting continuously unloaded and relaxed, is in constant work.

When you eat rarely, not often, you restore the work of your pancreas and your gallbladder. When you eat constantly, a certain amount of bile accumulates in your gallbladder and this process is permanent. This bile is used when you eat food, especially when you eat fatty and protein foods. When we eat 6-8-12 times a day, the gallbladder is working non-stop, and so we constantly lack bile.

For the entire history of evolution of its species, people have never eaten so much. Now, thanks to scientific and technical progress, we live in a civilization of food abundance. Eating so often is unnatural for humans and our digestive system.

Keep in mind, I'm not saying that you cannot slim down if you eat 6-8-12 times a day, as long as you are in a calorie deficit. However, if you want the process to be more effective, rare meals will work better! Why look for a more complicated way when there is an easier one?

In order to begin weight loss, we need to narrow down the time for consuming food during the day. You do not need to eat 12-14 hours during the day. It is just too much - we constantly eat, have high sugar levels in the blood, and it stops fat burning. Gradually over time, we need to reduce this eating time period down to 8 hours. For example, at first you can limit yourself to 12 hours. Then limit yourself to 10 hours. Then try 8 hours.

Step by step within a few weeks, you will get used to not eating immediately in the morning, and shift breakfast time a little bit later to spend calories first. This is especially important considering the fact that in the morning we have low blood sugar, and subsequently low insulin. Therefore, we have a good rate of fat burning.

The main task is to keep within this period of 8-9 hours. What for? So the remaining 16 hours your body will be without food, hence, the sugar level of your body will be low, and then insulin will be low. As soon as insulin falls, lipolysis begins. Once you have eaten something - high insulin stops any lipolysis.

What if it's difficult for you to limit your meal time to 8-9 hours throughout the day? It happens very often. This only means that the new food intake schedule is too different from what you have been used too previously. People who eat rarely get used to such a scheme easier than bodybuilders who usually eat very often. In order to eat food for only 8-9 hours a day, you need to gradually reduce the time of eating.

Let's say that your usual diet includes breakfast at 8.00 am and dinner at 11.00 pm. That means you eat 15 hours a day! And you need 8-9 hours!

What is better - to have dinner earlier or to have breakfast later? If you reduce the time of eating during the day, you will have to solve this problem. You can squeeze or stretch this eating period of time in both directions: both in the evening and in the morning. It depends on your individual schedule (work/study and training). My favorite time is the middle of the day. For example, I wake up at 7 am. In this case my first meal is often at 9-10 am, and the last meal at 6 pm.

If you have an evening workout (for example, at 7 pm), then try to shift your meals so that you take the last one in the evening (at 8-9 pm). In this case, your "breakfast" will move to lunch time. If you don't eat in the morning, the fat burns really fast because of the low blood sugar level.

I guess you understand now that you can actually eat in the evening. The most important thing is that you are limited to 8-9 hours in a day. This is a "time corridor" during which you can eat. It's not as difficult as it seems, but your mood and feelings will change dramatically, and the level of fat burning will substantially increase. There are 100% proven modern scientific data and experiments that can act as evidence for the nutrition program that I am now telling you about now.

If you eat healthy, not fatty and not sugary food, and also use a time limit for food intake, then you will achieve the maximum results. This mode of nutrition causes the greatest fat burning and the best physical condition with the ideal fat/dry weight ratio. Also, with this diet that you have the most chance of gaining muscle. A diet limited in time by 8-9 hours contributes much more to setting your balance between fat and dry body weight than all other diets that we usually use.

You may see how many people around you suffer from obesity. The more access we get to delicious, sweet, fat food, the fewer healthy people we see. This food, as well as unlimited access to it throughout the day, is actually killing us. This is the key reason that makes us gain weight and ruin our health.

Those of you who want to use this diet plan - do not be shy, you're welcome to leave comments about your results and health. I feel good, I'm in a good shape, I feel that my digestion improved and my strength did not decrease at all. I do not see any flaws in this scheme. At first I thought that I would have a certain hunger. However, there is no such side effects at all. You feel light inside. In the evening I have high performance – I'm always busy reading, doing something. I noticed that I used to feel the urge to eat something before. Now there is some sort of control, I can go get some water instead.

This is a certain manifestation of strength. Maybe the popular scheme that we constantly read about in bodybuilding magazines, that says we should eat 8 times a day, is not that effective after all. Recent scientific studies have shown that a 9-hour restriction in the intake of food does not harm your muscles, overall body composition, or health. Moreover, the efficiency of your muscles and stamina will double.

Just take a minute to think about the information that you've received. Everything you need to get rid of subcutaneous fat is at your fingertips, you can improve your condition, your health and even increase the efficiency of your muscles and stamina at the same time. No need for any terrible methods, no calorie counting - nothing complicated is needed. You just have to limit your time of eating in the day. You will look drier, and you will be healthier.

Thus, the second eating habit you must form is a "time corridor". Pay attention - you can eat as much as you want. At the first stage, we learned to eat the right foods and fewer wrong ones. At the second stage, you eat these right foods in a certain period of time. These two steps already lead us to indirectly create a calorie deficit, that is the basis of any weight loss plan that aims to get rid of subcutaneous fat.

It's likely that you will already begin to lose weight for long periods by implementing just these two levels. It is just forming a new eating habit and should be quite comfortable. You can eat as much as you want - but certain foods in a certain amount of time. Your body and brain are gradually going to become accustomed to it. You do not perceive this as suffering, or as some kind of stress. You have enough time to get used to the new diet gradually.

If, for some reason, the first 2 steps do not work, then it's only in the third stage that we begin to reduce the size of portions - the amount of right food to which we got used to eating at the first level. Getting rid of subcutaneous fat by limiting the incoming calories is much easier than at the expense of physical activity, exercise or cardio.

Step 3.

What do you need for the third stage? This is the honestly the most difficult part of your new eating plan because it requires cutting daily calories via actively reducing the amount of food. I advise you to go to this stage only after you have already got used to a solid diet (the first step) with limited meal times (second step).

If you cannot or don't want to change the time of food intake during the day by force of circumstances (your health/work schedule), then you need to go to the third step straight after step one.

Step 3 requires the cutting down of food in our diet very slowly to increase the calorie deficit, which is necessary to get rid of subcutaneous fat. In addition, we do not achieve this by sight, but under weekly controls and corrections.

Why do we count calories on a diet? I thought about this question once and found the answer: in order to grasp full control over the deficit needed for weight loss. As we all remember, the basic principle of any diet is to consume less energy than we expend every day. This is usually called a calorie deficit. So, in order to drop some weight, you need to make sure that you receive less calories than you spend on energy.

Why do people worry more about the amount of calories they eat rather than the amount and of food? The answer is very simple: people do not have the habit of eating the same set of foods in the same amount. Usually people eat spontaneously. Every day they eat different foods and in different amounts. In this context, one can only control the incoming energy by weighing all the food we eat and count the incoming calorie content according to online tables and calculators. However, this is not our situation. At the first stage, we left the harmful food aside and came about the right eating patterns. When people remove fatty and sugary foods, they suddenly notice they will subconsciously eat the same foods over and over again and even in the same amount.

So, if you eat according to our plan, you don't need to assess caloric intake. It is enough to just control and modify the usual amount of food.

What is the advantage of this method? Judge for yourself:

- You do not need to use measuring cups, glasses and other kitchen utensils.

- You do not have to bother about weighing foods on scales.

- You do not need to calculate calories from foods.

- You do not need to eat the same thing every day.

If we add carbohydrates or fats, then we gain mass, and if we reduce carbohydrates or fats, we lose weight. I recommend cutting carbohydrates, because I have noticed that people tend to overeat them easier when compared to fats. However, it is undesirable to remove carbohydrates completely, because this can slow down the fat burning in the long run.

How do I know how much food to cut out? To do this, you will need to monitor your body weight once a week. Remember, your weight should not decrease faster than 500-1000 g (1.1–2.2lb) in a week.

Here's what you should do every week:

- Weigh yourself once a week at the same time. Ideally straight out of bed, before eating and drinking, and after the toilet – this reduces the chance of weight fluctuations throughout the day.

- If your weight has not changed over the past week, then reduce carbohydrates by 1/8. Mind that you do not need to do this if your body shape is OK for you.

- If you dropped 500-1000 g (1.1–2.2lb), then do not change the diet for the next week.

- If you lost more weight during the past week, then raise the previous amount of carbohydrates in your diet by ¼.

How to restore the metabolic rate on a low-carb diet?

One of the reasons why the metabolism slows down on a low carbohydrate level is a decrease in the level of leptin that is produced in your system. Leptin is the satiety hormone secreted by fat tissue. The more leptin there is in your body, the more it suppresses your appetite. If you eat a lot, then the level of leptin is high. If you are on a diet, then the level of leptin is low and you constantly want to eat.

One of the most important functions of leptin is its effect on energy metabolism in our body. We start a diet to expend more energy than we consume with food every day. So, energy consumption and food intake depend on the concentration of leptin directly, as well as how all these processes are controlled from the hypothalamus. If you are on a strict diet, then the leptin concentration decreases very often, which leads to a metabolism and fat burning 'slowdown'.

Leptin has very diverse functions to slow down fat burning in your body. First of all, it effects your central nervous system through the hypothalamus which inevitably slows down all the processes of the metabolism. However, this is not all. Leptin affects the pancreas, kidneys, immune and sympathetic nervous system.

Here are some effects of leptin if there is a lot of it in your body:

- Increased energy consumption (rapid fat burning)

- Increased feeling of satiety (less food - no hunger)

- Reduced insulin secretion (food transport hormone)

- Increased diuresis (this is what bodybuilders do before competitions)

- Increased expression of growth factors (muscle growth)

- Stimulation of the immune system (people are often sick on a diet because of reduced immunity)

- Stimulation of bone growth and density (a hungry child may have rickets)

We can continue the list, but it's already clear that leptin plays a key role in the effectiveness of your diet. When there's enough leptin - you lose weight (usually the first 2-4 weeks of your diet). When leptin decreases - you starve and it shuts down your fat burning.

Similar to this, you may often see tips such as working out in order to "crank up your metabolism" on a diet. Right? One of the main mechanisms of this effect is that power (or speed) loading activates the leptin signal system in your muscles. As a result, there is a slight increase in energy consumption, which we perceive as a metabolism boost.

- Eating = Increasing leptin (feeling full)

- Hunger = Decrease in leptin (you want to eat)

- A lot of body fat = increase in leptin (fat people lose weight easily at the beginning)

- Low body fat = Decreased leptin (the most difficult last 5-10kg/11-22lb when drying out)

- Lots of insulin = Increased leptin (if you eat carbohydrates)

- Insulin is low = Decreased leptin (if you are on a low-carb diet)

- Cold = Decreased leptin (summer fat burning is easier)

As you can see, the main factor dictating the reduction in the level of leptin is food, carbohydrates, and insulin in particular. As soon as the body registers a regular decrease in the level of leptin on a diet, energy expenditure begins to slow down and the feeling of hunger increases. With regular training in the gym, this feeling only heightens.

A nutritional protocol known as a "carb refeed" is a way of eating that helps to cope with negative factors related to low leptin levels and slow energy expenditure.

The main idea of a refeed is that you have infrequent days with an increased carbohydrate intake in order to favorably stimulate ideal leptin production. Specifically, you increase the amount of carbohydrates by 50-100% every 4-30 days – the leaner you get, the more often you should refeed.

How often you should add refeeds to your diet depends on your health condition and shape. What does such a diet give us? Here are the reasons to give carb refeeds a shot:

- Increased energy expenditure – A temporary increase in carbohydrate intake can increase energy levels and allow more calories to be burned during both exercise and non-exercise induced activity.

- Reducing hunger – When you eat carbohydrates the amount of leptin produced will increase. This will give you a feeling of satiety and make further dieting easier (this is one of its main functions).

- Preservation of muscles - Insulin, produced in response to carbohydrate food, counteracts the increase in catabolism that is often heightened when losing weight (saves them).

- Improved well-being and appearance – The increase in carbohydrate intake will replenish glycogen stores in muscle tissue which is a key factor in looking 'full'.

Refeed VS Cheat meal

Why is a refeed better than a typical cheat meal? That's because cheat meals deceive your mind, not your metabolism. Cheat meals look goofy for me. It is common for athletes to load up on unhealthy food once per week all whilst giving it some scientific excuse. I understand why they do it. It is mentally difficult to be constantly restricted both in calories and in carbs. So people wait for the weekend, as some kind of celebration, hoping to indulge in mindless eating. This desire only arises because leptin levels fall. So, when the weekend comes, the athlete starts overeating and giving zero thought to what is being quickly put down their throats.

When refeeding, you control the leptin level and the quality of food you eat. With a cheat meal you do not control leptin (you go from a slight energy deficit, into a crazy high surplus, without any stability). In addition, cheat meals typically include cheeseburgers, pizza, etc. You eat bad foods in the amount that wouldn't be good for your health and for your muscles, in particular.

Conclusion: to correct the metabolic rate (leptin concentration) on a low-carb diet, it is necessary to incorporate a refeed every 4 days to several weeks. You don't need to eat a lot of cheat meals to crank up your weight loss. This doesn't work to speed up the metabolism, and is a big myth of nutrition.

Do not forget about sleep and wakefulness! Try to plan your day so that you are already in bed by 11 pm. There's an inextricable link between healthy sleep and a good physique.

• Sleep maintains a stable level of cortisol and a lack of sleep increases the stress hormone production that destroys muscle tissue (cortisol). It also transports fats to the abdominal area. During periods of stress, the level of this hormone is very high. Any diet, any shortage of calories is already a huge stress for your body. Sleep helps ease the tension. According to studies, people who lack sleep have higher cortisol levels in the daytime and early in the evening compared to those who sleep normally.

•   Sleep controls the blood glucose level. Have you ever noticed that a night without sleep is always followed by over-eating? According to American scientists, the lack of sleep affects the metabolism and hormonal system, entailing a number of endocrine and metabolic disorders. Signs of this process are hunger and fatigue which our body perceives as a signal for saving and storing energy. Researchers also noted that a lack of sleep reduces your glucose level and insulin sensitivity, which are essential in preventing diabetes.

•   The effectiveness and intensity of your workouts also depends on sleep length and quality. Any body transformation depends upon recovery. Weight loss, recovery from illness, restoration of damaged muscle tissue all occurs mainly during sleep. Without recovering, you cannot work out effectively. Therefore, it is essential to provide yourself with sufficient rest which will help not only help to increase the effectiveness of training, which ultimately fine-tunes your results, but also to control appetite, give clarity of mind, and become an invaluable contribution to health.

What should I do to sleep well?

A healthy sleep is equally important for weight loss and growth. Therefore, if tomorrow you want to become better than today, try these tips:

1. Avoid caffeine in the evening - > 3 hours from going to bed).

2. Do not exercise late at night - Finish your workout at least 45 minutes before bedtime.

3. Do not drink a lot of water before going to bed - It takes about

an hour to get rid of excess fluid so you can sleep through the night.

4. Learn to go to bed at the same time even on weekends.

5. Do not sleep too much in the daytime - A 20-30 minute nap is enough to stimulate recovery.

6. Find your favorite position for sleep - If you place the pillow under your feet, this will relieve back tension, and if you like to sleep on your side, then try putting a pillow between your legs for more comfort and support for your hips.

7. Use pillows of the correct size.

8. Sleep in complete darkness - turn off the light, close the curtains, cover the lights from electronic devices, or even better, disconnect them.

9. Eat protein foods (chicken, cottage cheese, eggs, yogurt) for dinner – They contain the amino acid tryptophan that is important for sound sleep.

Step 4.

The fourth step deals with your physical activity. When I talk about physical activity, I mean:

• Everyday activities necessary for your daily routine (travelling to work, to the store, home, studying, etc.). Any non-training specific activity.

• Training activity includes any training involving your osteomuscular system. There are two major directions here: anaerobic (gym, power work) activity and aerobic (running, walking, orbitrack, etc.) activity.

What is the main idea of step 4? You need to increase the amount of energy that you spend on any form of physical activity during the day. We followed our diet closely during steps 1-3 and didn't think about training and basic activity in general (so most likely it wasn't optimal during this time). Now it's time to fix it.

Is it possible to avoid the 4th stage? It is, if you have achieved the desired percentage of subcutaneous fat and don't want to change your body any further. However, it is easier to achieve the desired result by forming both the correct eating patterns and by using physical activity. Therefore, the 4th stage is not mandatory if you just want to lose weight.

Can we avoid additional training? Yes. However, consider two things. Power training helps retain muscle tissue during long periods with a limited calorie supply (so you look better) and increases your daily energy expenditure (so it's easier to melt fat). In addition, aerobic exercise has a direct effect on your subcutaneous fat as stored fat will be used as an energy source to fuel this type of activity.

How do I go over to the 4th stage in practice?

•   If you have never exercised, then you need to start going to the gym.

•   If you used to only go to the gym, then you need to add interval training cardio.

•   If you used to only do cardio, then you need to add power training.

•   If you already do cardio and power training, then you need to adjust them according to your goals and the amount of food that you consume every day.

In practice, this is done by an increase/decrease in the frequency and time of training.

The main reason for what is commonly deemed as a "slowing metabolism" from dieting is actually an unconscious decrease in non-exercise induced activity – this contains all types of sub-conscious movement, such as walking to the kitchen, taking the stairs, or even talking speed! Yes, this will effect your fat burning over time, as your body will subconsciously choose 'easier' and less energy-consuming tasks when in an energy deficit from diet and/or training.

I recommend controlling your daily activity, not training activity. Training activity is what you do in the gym. This is activity you do to lose weight, and it burns a small amount of calories compared to non-exercise induced activity. Despite what trainers in the gyms tell you – you don't burn too many calories in the gym relative to the entirety of the day.

Household chores and other daily activities are more important because during workouts you consciously control your energy consumption (minutes, approaches, reps, speed, etc.) and training time is limited to 30-60 minutes, while the rest of the time - it's your usual daily activity (more important).

There is a peculiarity of our bodies proved by numerous experiments: if we're on a diet, calories burn more slowly. As a rule, pseudo-specialists explain this by a slow down of the metabolism. This is complete nonsense, many experiments have proved it. For example, the Minnesota hungry experiment showed that the expenditure of calories actually slows down, but not because of a slowing metabolism (it hardly weakens), but due to the fact that a person unconsciously starts moving less and saving energy – this is a survival mechanism during old times of starvation for energy preservation purposes.

If you learn to control your everyday physical activity, you'll be able to consciously increase it. For example, don't drive to the store, just walk - a kilometer to the store and back.

You will get much greater results using these simple tricks than from any workout at a gym.

If you want to directly melt off your subcutaneous fat, you should practice exercising at a low intensity - walking, fast walking or very slow jogging. I usually walk fast.

You should change your daily routine to increase everyday activity – I'm talking about adding something more to your usual actions. For example, you can adjust your schedule in such a way that you get to work on a bicycle or walk there. At work, you can squat or do push-ups every 2 hours (if this is permitted and possible at your work, of course). You do not change checkpoints (common tasks), but you are changing activity in the process of achieving them. The goal is to add activity to your usual daily routine.

Let's now talk about training activity. Namely, about aerobic and anaerobic training to achieve the desired results.

How do aerobic and anaerobic exercises differ:

•   Aerobic activities are low-intensity, requiring oxygen, fat and carbohydrate reserves for energy supply (for example, running, walking, bicycling, swimming and other types of cyclic activity).

•   Anaerobic activities are high-intensity, and don't require oxygen for energy supply, so carbohydrates are utilised in the form of glycogen stores for energy use (this refers to any power training from bodybuilding to weightlifting or shot put).

The most important difference between these two types of training activity is that during anaerobic activity it is predominantly glycogen (carbohydrates) that is burnt, whereas it is mainly fat that is burnt during aerobic activity. On the other hand, anaerobic exercises are more effective at sustaining an increased burning of calories outside of exercise, in contrast to aerobic exercise. In addition, power (anaerobic) training helps to retain muscle tissue during a diet. To make it clear, here are the main consequences of each type of training:

Aerobic exercise (cardio):

•	Oxidation of fatty acids (direct burning of fat in small amounts)

•	Increased blood circulation (by increasing the number of capillaries)

•	Increase in the number of mitochondria and fat-burning enzymes

•	Transformation of glycolytic ("power") fibers into oxidative ("endurance") fibers.

•	Reduction of energy consumption at rest (energy efficiency is increased)

Anaerobic exercise (power):

•	Increase in oxygen consumption (after exercise)

•	Increase in total energy expenditure (through the expenditure of glycogen and other mechanisms)

•	Increase in the amount of glycogen in the muscles and corresponding enzymes

•	Increased muscular efficiency

•   Transformation of oxidative ("endurance") fibers into glycolytic ("power") fibers.

As you can see, these two types of activities contradict each other. The more you work out at the gym, the less endurance you have while running. The more you run, the smaller and weaker your muscles become. What should we do then? What kind of physical activity should we choose?

I believe that if you aim for a good (lean) body, and not a gain of the maximum possible amount of muscle mass, then you need to use these two types together. The power training will conserve your muscle mass, increase strength, and total energy consumption. At the same time, aerobic exercises will give you direct fat burning, glucose disposal, improved endurance and cardiovascular health.

By the way, the utilization of glucose is a very important parameter for fat burning, because the faster the utilization is, the lower the blood sugar will be and the more lipolysis is activated. Meanwhile, despite the fact that power training greatly increases the total energy expenditure both during and after training, it practically does not accelerate the utilization of glucose.

Thus, for maximum fat burning, two types of workouts work better than power training alone.

Which cardio burns body fat better?

If we talk about the long-term perspective (calories burnt over a whole day, not just in the gym), then high-intensity exercises (very fast running) work better, but if you need fat burning "here and now", then low-intensity training (fast walking) works better.

•   The higher the training intensity is, the more glycogen and less fat is burnt.

•   The lower the intensity is, the more fat and less glycogen is burnt.

But:

•   The higher the intensity is, the greater the subsequent (post-exercise) energy expenditure is.

•   The lower the intensity is, the lower the subsequent (post-exercise) energy expenditure is.

As you can see, we have a contradiction. Pros in one direction create cons in the other. To make it more clear consider three examples:

• walking 5 kph (3.1 mph) = - 5 kcal/min. (fat = 100%)

• running 10 kph (6.2 mph) = - 10 kcal/min. (fat = 50% + glycogen = 50%)

• fast running 15 kph (9.3 mph) = - 15 kcal/min. (glycogen = 100%)

As you can see low-intensity cardio (walking) only burns fat, and high-intensity cardio (fast running) only burns glycogen (carbohydrates). However, when you deplete the stores of glycogen, there is an increase in the oxidation of fats. In addition, high-intensity cardio (fast running or power training) causes more energy expenditure than low-intensity cardio.

So how should we run? It depends on your goals ⌐and physique. If you want to lose weight in any way possible without paying attention to waste (muscle and strength reduction), then you can do high-intensity cardio. However, if you want to save your muscles, and you don't really need a very fast result, then it's better to do low-intensity cardio.

What if you use interval running? If you accelerate really fast, then consider that this is purely high-intensity training, i.e. only glycogen will burn.

How to increase the direct burning of fat (not glycogen)? I want to share the ideas of Professor Seluyanov. We all haven't got quite the right idea about how to do cardio to get rid of subcutaneous fat. It is usually believed that the more, the better. Usually it is considered that it is necessary to run for at least an hour. If you are a crazy fan – people say it will be better if you run for 2-3 hours.

This scheme works, but there is a very serious flaw in it, which we do not take into account. We constantly confuse subcutaneous fat and intramuscular fat. Indeed, anaerobic oxidation of fat occurs during exercise. We walk, and walk, and walk and fat from under our skin gradually burns out. When we do low-intensity cardio, it burns out the intramuscular fat, says Prof. Siluanov. Not the subcutaneous fat!

Subcutaneous fat cannot burn during aerobic training, it cannot be wasted. You might object to that: how come, I tried low-intensity cardio, I'm losing weight with it! The reason is that there is a constant migration of subcutaneous fat into the intramuscular in that situation, if you have created a calorie deficit. So you do low-intensity cardio, and then you activate anaerobic oxidation of fat, which is in our muscles - intramuscular fat. Then it is wasted. And then what? It is actively wasted if you create the right conditions – exercise from thirty to fifty minutes. Then you need: 1) either to stop your workout, because you have spent all your intramuscular fat and depleted its reserves, or 2) arrange re-interval cardio - this means to have the same amount of rest after the training session as compared with the duration of the training session. That is, if you have been walking or running at a low pace for half an hour - then relax, sit down, and read something for half an hour! While you rest, the exhausted stocks of intramuscular fat will be replenished by subcutaneous fat. This is what we need!

When there is a deficit in our body, the subcutaneous fat constantly migrates into the intramuscular fat. If we want to constantly melt it, then we need to cause this movement from subcutaneous fat to intramuscular. To do this, we need to rest between low-intensity training sessions. That is, if we walk at a fast pace for half an hour or fifty minutes, we also rest for the same amount of time. Fat from under our skin becomes intramuscular. Again walking, then resting. Such a re-interval cardio allows you to significantly improve the effectiveness of your training. Fat will burn, real fat! It is very important not to consume carbs during the rest periods because it will inhibit the important process of lipolysis - fat burning. Re-interval cardio is not my idea, it's Professor Siluanov's. I just decided to share it, because it works well.

The idea of Seluyanov's method is that in order to burn off subcutaneous fat, it first has to split into glycerin and fatty acids. The latter should get into muscles and be used as an energy source during low-intensity cardio. The professor believes that after you expend these fatty acids, you need to rest for 30-50 minutes, so that a new portion of fat can be oxidized and ready to be used by muscle cells.

This is the ideal training scheme by Seluyanov:

• 30-50 minutes of cardio (fast walking or jogging). Fatty acids burn in the muscles.

• 30-50 minutes of rest (no activity, no food). Fats are oxidized to fatty acids.

• 30-50 minutes of cardio (fast walking or jogging). Fatty acids burn in the muscles.

• 30-50 minutes of rest (no activity, no food). Fats are oxidized to fatty acids.

I myself used this method before and still use it now, for example, while walking with a baby stroller around the park. While my baby sleeps, I walk with a stroller for 30 minutes, then rest on the bench for the same amount of time. You can literally feel your fat burning! This requires minimal effort, no long intensive workout needed. This is what we call a modern scientific approach.

I understand that it is unlikely that you will do cardio for half a day on such a scheme. However, this is not required. You can break a 60-minute cardio for 30 minutes in the morning and 30 minutes in the evening. The most important thing is that you understand this principle - "after fatty acids are consumed it takes the same amount of time to make them available for expenditure again."

If you've never worked out properly at the gym before, then I recommend that you take up the "full body" program three times a week - training the whole body, all muscle groups, in one workout. This means that you will work on all the main muscles on your body in each workout. Here is an example of such a program for a beginner:

- Squats with a barbell on shoulders 4 X 10

- Pull-ups 4 x as many as possible

- Bench Press / on an incline bench 4 X 10

- Dumbbell presses standing or sitting 4 x 10

Only 'working sets' are listed. First there should be several warm-ups with light weights.

The first time you complete a gym session you will undoubtably have muscle aches within 24-48 hours. Due to this, they will likely not have enough time to "heal" for the next workout. However, it is important to know that this process of inadequate recovery will end within a month because your muscles will adapt to the load and stress.

What is the best time to work out? It's scientifically proved that:

•   The best time for cardio workout and fat burning is in the morning

•   The best time for power training is in the evening

It's cool if you have two workouts (morning and evening). The ideal situation is cardio and power training on different days.

What if you want to do two types of training at once? In this case, start with a cardio load, and then do the power. There is a popular strategy to do cardio after strength training in order to achieve better fat burning on the basis that you will have lower blood sugar. Unfortunately, this strategy is very bad for the muscles (during cardio all growth factors are destroyed) and not that good for fat burning (according to a number of experiments). In general, first we run, then we push and pull the weights.

Women and men also have different energy supplies during and after training. There is a certain imbalance in carbohydrates and fats in different periods:

• MEN = during the training session GLYCOGEN (carbs) is used / after the training - FAT

• WOMEN = during the training FAT (less carbs) / after - GLYCOGEN

This does not mean that women use little glycogen during a

power or other high-intensity workout. They use it, but to a lesser extent than men. However, after training (during recovery) everything changes. The female body starts to use carbohydrates well, while the male body opts mainly for fatty acids. Perhaps this phenomenon is related to the fact that there are more red (endurance) muscle fibers in the female body that oxidize fatty acids well because of the large number of mitochondria that is present. To make it very simple, women need less carbohydrates and glycogen than men. Especially if we are talking about losing weight.

Is local fat burning possible? There is one popular myth about local fat burning. Say, if you do a lot of sit-ups, you can supposedly burn more fat specifically over your ab region. It's a lie. Local reduction of fat is not possible!

This means that when a person starts off a diet, he/she loses fat in all areas, not in some certain one. Here we need to stop and take a look into physiology. Fat is stored in cells (liposomes) in a substance called triglycerides. Under the influence of two stress hormones (adrenaline and noradrenaline) the splitting of fat cells into glycerin and fatty acids begins. This is called lipolysis. The substances obtained begin their journey through the bloodstream until they are disposed of, or, if they are not needed any longer, they return to their original state (fat). Now you understand that fat splitting is a chemical reaction in its pure form, which is triggered by hormones. They travel through blood that "washes" our whole body. It is not possible to force the blood to come only to your abs and so it is not possible to force the hormones to break down fat in only one place where it's desirable for you.

In general, this topic causes a hotly contested debate every time. For example, there is an opinion that the increase in blood flow in a certain place of your body contributes to the "washing" of this place with catecholamines. However, numerous experiments show that fat does not burn locally.

For example, in one of sciences recent experiments, people isolated and only trained ... one leg. This was done for the purpose to find out if local fat burning, or something similar, exists. Later, scientists measured the levels of fat in the trained and not trained leg. Guess what they found? Decreased fat on their whole body, but no significant difference in the amount of fat burnt in each separate leg.

The bottom-line is: local fat burning is impossible. There's no need to do extra sets and reps of exercises on the part of your body where you would most like to melt fat.

CONCLUSION

So, let's take a look through the main steps again.

Step 1 = remove "bad" (sweet, fatty) foods. Get used to eating the right foods every day.

Step 2 = gradually reduce the time eating period during the day (up to 8-9 hours) and get used to this schedule of eating.

Step 3 = reduce the amount of food per day using your initiative (and not calories) for food intake control. Landmark - weight loss of 0.5-1 kg per week (1.1-2.2lb).

Step 4 = add and control physical activity throughout the day. This is primarily focused towards non-training induced exercise and regular day-to-day activities. Training activity should take second place, although this is also important.

ATTENTION! Your goal is to form the right eating habit. Losing weight is an intermediate (not the main) goal. Give yourself as much time as you need to master every new step. It usually takes 1-2 months to get used to something new. If possible, do not jump over steps. Do not start using all the steps at once. Otherwise, sooner or later, you will return to mindless eating as you will not properly adapt to each step and progress as needed. The way people look shows their attitude to themselves. The bottom line is that by dropping fat, you will achieve a new attitude to yourself, to life, and to other people.

You need to go through these four stages gradually – step by step, giving as much time as you need for each step, giving time to your body to get used each protocol. Unfortunately, your interests are opposed to the interests of the fitness industry. As a smart person, you want a long-term result - to get a sexy, slim, fat-free body for good. The fitness industry is not interested in this, because with this scenario they will not be able to earn money from you. It's one thing if you lose some weight, get the result, then gain weight again – and so you spend hard-earned money to lose weight over and over again. It's a completely different thing when you receive a permanent life-long result, and you do not need to buy fat burners, you do not need to buy a gym membership, pay coaches and so on. The entire fitness industry is interested in your temporary result, so that you put on weight and become fat again. At each of these stages they can earn money from you.

Now you know about the benefits of good habits, now you know that if you want a permanent result - you need to form the right eating patterns. Most importantly - the restrictions should be very small and gradual. The speed with which you are getting to the result is not important. It is just important that you are consistently moving in the right direction. You will gain control over your physique, over the percentage of fat on your body, and you will look good.

All the tools described in this material are very effective for shredding fat off your body. If you do everything the way it is written here, your life will significantly change. It's not only that you will look good and feel great. The fact is that you will receive a unique experience of control over the situation, which will give you a new-found pleasure and confidence. In general, for my part, I did everything I needed. You now understand what you need to do. Your move…